The Ketogenic Diet

The Secret to Weight Loss Revealed

The Beginners Guide to Fitness and Weight Loss while On the Ketogenic Diet

Omar Peart

I0441313

The Ketogenic Diet

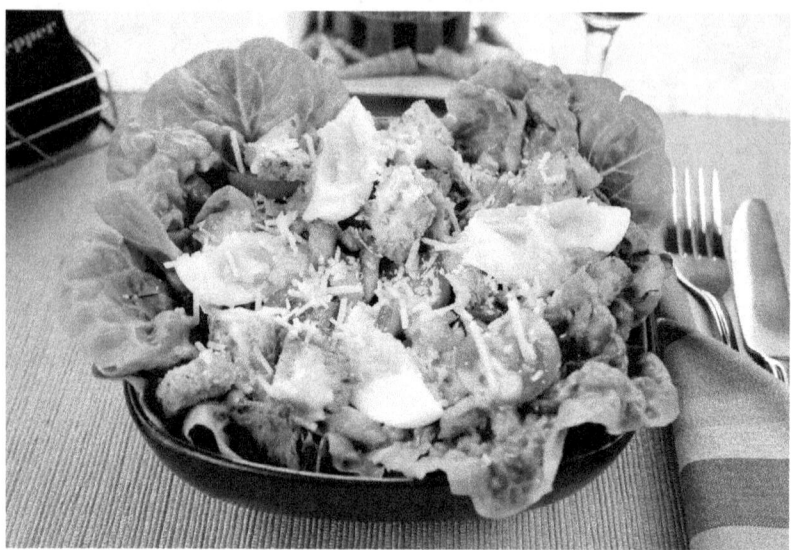

Omar Peart

COPYRIGHT

We support copyright of all intellectual property. Copyright protection continues to spark the seed of creativity in content producers, ensures that everyone has their voice heard through the power of words and the captivity of a story. Uniqueness of culture and content has been passed down through generations of storytelling and is the DNA of every intelligent species on our planet.

FINDING THE PERFECT DIET...

If you are struggling to lose weight and you have tried all the diets that you can think of do not despair. There is a diet out there that has helped many people to lose the excess weight. It is the ketogenic diet. It has been around for years and it has made its resurgence in the past few years as the benefits of being on such a diet are discovered by more persons.

Why Omar Wrote This Book...

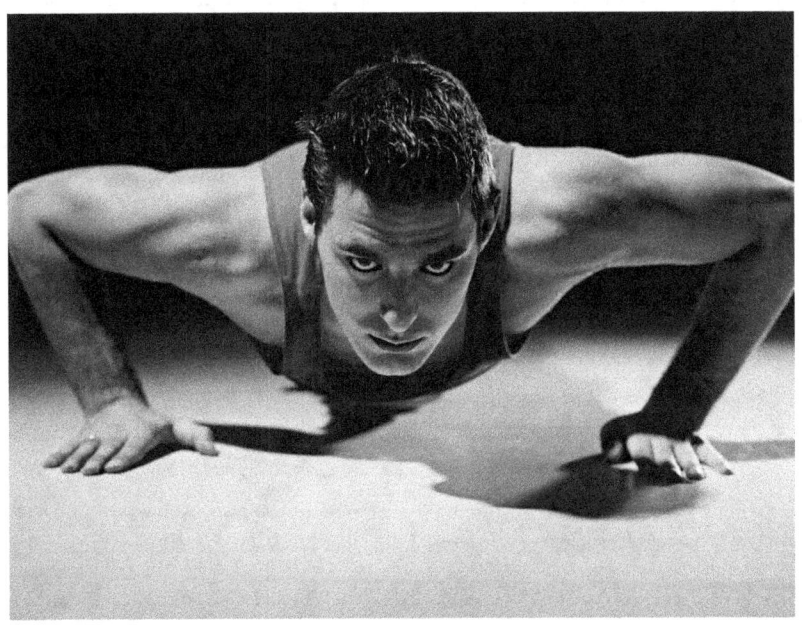

OMAR PEART IS A NON-FICTION WRITER and has written books on a myriad of topics. He has a love for health and wellness and as such he spends a lot of time researching diets and sharing the information that he has found with others through his books.

Omar has been on his own personal journey with weight loss and he has found one diet in particular, the ketogenic diet to be beneficial to his needs. His latest book focuses on that. He shares the advantages and disadvantages of the diet, leaving the reader to make an informed decision. He also includes some great bonus recipes at the end for all to try.

TABLE OF CONTENTS

COPYRIGHT 3

FINDING THE PERFECT DIET… 4

WHY OMAR WROTE THIS BOOK… 5

GETTING HEALTHY 8

DEDICATION 9

WHAT YOU NEED TO KNOW ABOUT THE KETOGENIC DIET 10

So You Want To Try the Ketogenic Diet 10

Understanding What Ketosis Is 12

Ketoacidosis a Silent Killer.. 15

Diabetic Ketoacidosis.. 16

Alcoholic Ketoacidosis... 18

Causes of Ketoacidosis 19

Symptoms of Ketosis.. 21

THE ADVANTAGES AND DISADVANTAGES OF THE KETO DIET....................24

Advantages of a Ketogenic Diet.. 24

Disadvantages of the Ketogenic Diet 26

GETTING STARTED ON THE WEIGHT LOSS REGIME.....................................29

List 5 Ways You Can Motivate Yourself to Lose Weight.......................... 29

Exercise To Burn 1,000 Calories per Day and How to Do Them 31

EAT THIS NOT THAT – FOODS YOU NEED AND DON'T NEED ON THE KETO DIET 33

Eating Daily to Consume 1500 Calories.................................... 33

Eat These Superfoods That Help to Boost Metabolism and Weight Loss . 34

Good & Bad Fats 36

Benefits of Omega-3 Fatty Oils... 38

Fish & the Ketogenic Diet.. 39

Benefits of Eating Red and White Meat 41

Spinach and Kale – Essential Foods for the Ketogenic Diet...................... 43

Dairy Products Such As Cheese and Sour Cream Are Staple On the

Ketogenic Diet.. 45

Spices That Can Be Consumed When On a Ketogenic Diet 47

ONE MONTH OF KETOGENIC RECIPES 60

KETOGENIC DIET BREAKFAST RECIPES 61

Yogurt, Spinach, Chili Oil Baked Eggs 61

Tofu Scramble 63

Quinoa Breakfast 65

Bacon and Eggs 66

KETOGENIC DIET LUNCH RECIPES 67

Herbed Cheese and Tomato 67

Turkey Wrap 69

Grilled Turkey Sandwich with Cheese and Tomato 70

Bean Burrito 71

KETOGENIC DIET DINNER RECIPES 72

Arugula and Pear Salad Topped with Candied Walnuts (208 calories) 72

Chile Relleno Mini Casserole (215 calories) 73

Butternut Baja Squash Soup (55 calories) 75

Lettuce Leaf Tacos (550 calories) 77

KETOGENIC DIET VEGETABLE SMOOTHIE RECIPES 79

Beetroot Spinach Almond Smoothie 79

Beetroot Cherry Lettuce Smoothie 80

Topical Green Smoothie 81

Spinach Peach Smoothie 82

Cherry Cabbage Smoothie 83

Winter Blueberries Smoothie 84

Broccoli and Spinach Apple Smoothie 85

Cucumber Mint Smoothie 86

Asparagus Smoothie 87

Mango Spinach Honey Smoothie 88

GETTING HEALTHY

"A healthy outside starts from the inside."

Robert Urich

DEDICATION

"This book is dedicated to those who are seeking a solution to their dietary challenges. Finding the right solution can take time so it is important not to become too disappointed at the first try. The same diet that works for someone else may not work for you. I thank my mother for instilling that in me."

WHAT YOU NEED TO KNOW ABOUT THE KETOGENIC DIET

So You Want To Try the Ketogenic Diet

This is a special diet that is composed of high fat and low carbohydrate foods and is usually administered to people with epilepsy to help control their seizures. The diet is usually administered and monitored by dieticians through the provision of calories, fluids and proteins in careful measurements.

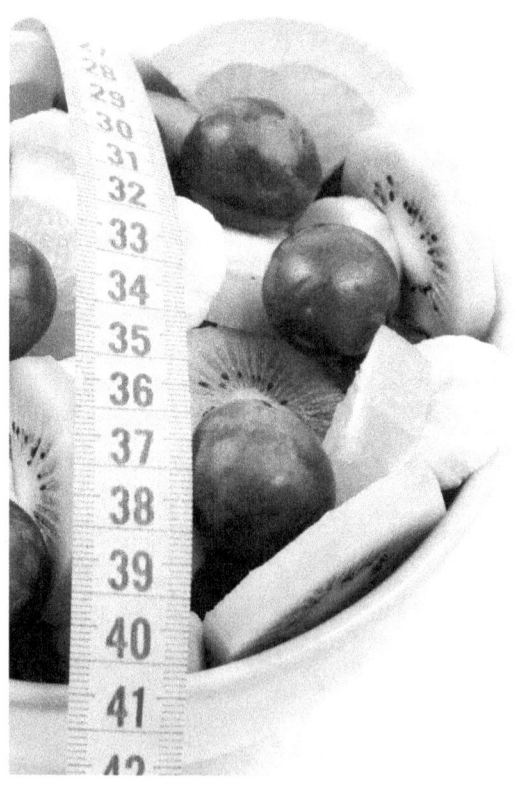

Omar Peart
History of the Ketogenic Diet

The ketogenic diet is believed to have been designed by Dr Russel Wilder around 1924 when he worked at the Mayo Clinic. The diet became popular as a way of treating seizures for patients with epilepsy but fell out of fashion around the 1940s due to the emergence of new anti seizures medication.

The Charlie Foundation was started in 1994 by Charlie Abraham's family after he used the ketogenic diet which helped him to fight off the seizures and lead a healthy and normal life.

What Is Contained In the Ketogenic Diet?

Carbohydrates

Ketogenic diets revolve around how much carbohydrates are consumed, an individual's metabolism rate and their activity level. For athletes with a healthy metabolism, it is acceptable for them to consume more than 100 grams of carbohydrates in a day.

For those who consume 50 to 60 grams of carbohydrates, their diet is automatically considered ketogenic.

Protein

Proteins are the building blocks in our bodies therefore it is important to maintain consumption of certain amount and avoid overdoing it to avoid going into the ketosis state. It is advisable to follow your physician's prescription regarding the consumption of proteins.

Fat

Fats are usually converted and utilized as fuel by the body when it is performing different functions. It is important to note that most calories in the diet usually originate from fats. Weight loss and other factors usually help one to determine how much calories they need to consume in a day. The physician will be able to prescribe the correct amount that one needs to consume in a day.

Understanding What Ketosis Is

Several ketones are at work in the human body, but some are concerning to medical professionals, and these are the ones produced through fat metabolism. These ketones are needed for cells in the body to provide energy. Our brains can use these ketones for nearly 75 percent of its energy requirements. Ketones are presumably generated under particular conditions:

When carbohydrate exists but the body is unable to use glucose, it is typically due to insufficient insulin, which is seen in Type 1 diabetes.

Generally, your body's mechanisms will stop ketones from reaching dangerously high levels. However, the last condition – unrelated to insulin – is known to allow ketone levels to spiral into dangerous levels and creating a condition known as ketoacidosis. Ketoacidoses may or may not be linked to insulin-related conditions, and is said to also appear during a diet of low carbohydrate ketogenic. Dieters will often monitor their ketone levels in an effort to avoid ketoacidosis.

Is Ketosis Dangerous?

Medical professionals define ketosis as potentially dangerous and a very serious condition.

Ketosis said to be dangerous as extremely high levels of ketones can cause the blood in your body to become acidic – ketoacidosis -- which can lead to severe illness in a very short time period.

The American Heart Association and the American Cancer Society, along with the National Cholesterol Education Program -- all agree that a diet that reduces calories from protein is the one to use.

Other conditions and illnesses related to ketosis include:

High Cholesterol

Osteoporosis and kidney stones

Kidney problems

Although ketosis is not the direct cause of the above illnesses and conditions; the root cause of ketosis and these conditions is equal. If ketosis is present in your body, then you should have these conditions monitored and tested as well.

Symptoms of ketosis:

Fatigue

Headache

Extreme thirst

Dry mouth

Bad breath: fruity and unpleasant

Metallic taste in your mouth

Faintness

Weak

Dizziness

Sleep problems

Nausea or stomachache

Cold hands and/or feet

Frequent urination

Ketoacidosis a Silent Killer

Ketoacidosis is more appropriately called diabetic ketoacidosis. It is caused when the body contains high levels of ketones due to accelerated natural production. Ketones are a particular type of blood acid that in high levels can affect the body adversely. The levels become high because of a body's inability to produce adequate amounts of insulin. Insulins most noted effect is in regulating a body's glucose levels.

A result of this deficiency of insulin is that a body begins to consume its own fat cells for energy, instead of the insulin regulated glucose that it would normally use to power a body's muscles and other tissues. This has the effect of causing a toxic buildup of very acidic ketones in the bloodstream. When this is allowed to fester untreated, the result is diabetic ketoacidosis. The onset of symptoms can happen very quickly, and this is sometimes the first signs of diabetes that a sufferer may experience.

Chronically untreated ketoacidosis can be fatal. In addition, it can cause low blood sugar and the complications that this condition facilitates. Low blood sugar is also called hypoglycemia and it is marked by swiftly decreasing blood sugar levels. It can also cause low potassium and the related issues. However, these are related to the treatments for diabetic ketoacidosis and low potassium can affect the heart and other muscle functions. When children first experience symptoms of this disease, the treatments can cause brain swelling if not applied properly. Brain swelling is called cerebral edema. This is the danger of diabetic ketoacidosis. Because it occurs as a precursor to diabetes, it may have gone untreated, and then the treatments can be as dangerous as the disease itself as both can be fatal. It is best that people familiarize themselves with the symptoms of diabetic ketoacidosis to prevent this disease from going undiagnosed. There are several over-the-counter testing kits for both hypoglycemia and diabetic ketoacidosis.

Diabetic Ketoacidosis

Diabetic Ketoacidosis (DKA) is a condition people with diabetes sometimes develop when their bodies lack the insulin necessary to process the glucose in their blood to provide the cells with the energy they need. The kidneys then begin filtering the sugar out of the blood and disposing of it through the urine.

As a result, the body begins to break down fat and muscle to use as fuel. One of the byproducts of this process is the creation of ketones. The buildup of these ketones inside the body leads to the life-threatening condition known as diabetic ketoacidosis.

Ketones are fatty-acids. When too many ketones enter the bloodstream, it can sometimes lead to a chemical imbalance called diabetic ketoacidosis. There are a number of reasons diabetics may develop ketoacidosis. Their blood sugar level may have gotten too high. They may have become severely dehydrated. The diabetic may have developed an infection or some other type of illness. Sometimes diabetic ketoacidosis develops because the body simply didn't produce enough insulin. Often the condition is caused by a combination of all those factors.

People with type 1 diabetes are highly susceptible to this condition. Type 2 diabetes sufferers, especially children, can sometimes develop the condition also. The symptoms of diabetic ketoacidosis include blurred vision, hot, flushed, dry skin, difficulty waking up or drowsiness, constantly feeling thirsty and urinating excessively, rapid, deep breathing, loss of appetite, stomach pains, vomiting, and confusion. If a diabetic develops these symptoms they can use ketone test strips or visit a hospital to have their blood and urine tested.

If the diabetic ketoacidosis is found to be severe, the person may require hospitalization and intensive care. The treatment normally entails administering insulin and other fluids and monitoring to ensure there is no swelling of the brain. The process of getting the blood sugar levels to normal may take several days of intensive treatment.

Alcoholic Ketoacidosis

Alcoholic ketoacidosis develops when ketones, a type of acid formed from the creation of energy by the breaking down of fat, build up in the blood. Excessive alcohol use causes this form of metabolic acidosis. It is most common in the malnourished that drink excessively because it results from a combination of alcoholism and starvation. Undernourishment can result because those that drink excessively might not eat properly.

Symptoms of Alcoholic Ketoacidosis include but are not limited to confusion, fatigue, sluggishness and a decreased level of alertness. There is a danger of coma if symptoms of sluggishness are too severe. There may also be a lack of appetite, thirst, dizziness and even vomiting. There are a number of blood tests and urine tests that are done in the event that alcoholic ketoacidosis may be present. Blood alcohol level and a toxicology screen may be performed. Measurement of blood clotting may be performed. Urine ketones and arterial blood gases may also be checked during the performance of various tests.

Treatments for alcoholic ketoacidosis include an intravenous solution of sugar and salt. Those suffering may be required to have their blood taken often and need nutritional supplements. The supplements are for the treatment of deficiencies resulting from excessive alcohol use. Hospital admission, typically to the intensive care unit, is usually required for the treatment of this condition. The prevention of withdrawals may be aided with additional medication.

Prompt medical attention is required to improve the prognosis although there are other factors that can affect the outcome of the disease. The severity of alcoholism, state of the liver and other complications or diseases will have an effect on the prognosis. Alcoholic ketoacidosis can be life threatening. Gastrointestinal bleeding, inflammation of the pancreas, seizures, coma and pneumonia are all potential complications. Those that drink excessively are at a higher risk for alcoholic ketoacidosis, limiting alcohol consumption can aid in the prevention of this disease.

Causes of Ketoacidosis

Here are the top 4 common causes of diabetic ketoacidosis.

1) Insulin Deficiency

Metabolism is a term that is used to describe the break down food within the body that gets converted into energy and nutrients. Insulin regulates the blood sugar levels of the body as it converts food into energy. Whenever there is a lack of insulin or if the body cannot utilize insulin efficiently, it will try to break down fat instead. Unfortunately, this breakdown of fat equates to the release of ketones which are acidic chemicals. This accumulation of acidic chemicals causes the body to release vast amounts of urine which can cause dehydration.

2) Infection

Another common cause for ketoacidosis is an infection. Whenever an infection occurs within the body, the body responds by increasing its glucose production rate. This accumulation of glucose can cause insulin treatment solutions to become ineffective, which in turn causes ketoacidosis. Some common infections that diabetics undergo which eventually trigger ketoacidosis are: pneumonia, influenza and gastroenteritis.

3) Delay in Diagnosis

While it may be true that the symptoms of type 1 diabetes may manifest itself relatively quickly, many people do not know what those specific symptoms may indicate. As such, they usually associate these symptoms with being sick and as such, never contemplate about the possibility of being screened for diabetes until they realize that the symptoms are not going away. During this type period, without sufficient insulin treatment solution, the condition may have already progressed to ketoacidosis.

4) Lifestyle Choices

One of the most common reasons why diabetics experience ketoacidosis, is due to the consumption of drugs and substances that causes their insulin levels to decrease. Illegal drugs such as cocaine, ketamine, ecstasy, heroin and methadone can deplete the body's level of insulin. It's also worth noting that binge drinking can deplete the body's level of insulin as well.

Some other causes of ketoacidosis include:

Stroke

Heart attack

Damaged insulin pump

Psychological stress

Potassium deficiency

Symptoms of Ketosis

When a very low-carbohydrate diet is consumed for several days, people suffering from ketosis may experience the following symptoms:

Breath that smells fruity or like nail polish remover; this occurs as the body eliminates excess ketones through the lining of the lungs.

An increase in the frequency of urination, which is the body's attempt to flush out extra ketones in the urine- Unfortunately, this can also significantly reduce levels of key electrolyte minerals like sodium, potassium and magnesium. Many experts recommend increasing your intake of these minerals by drinking broth and eating mineral-rich vegetables.

Dry mouth caused by increased urination. Drinking more water can help to relieve this symptom.

Headache, which is causes by a lack of carbohydrates and may be worsened by dehydration and low electrolytes.

Fatigue and low energy- This symptom results from the body lacking carbohydrates to convert into energy. As the body becomes used to burning fat for energy, this issue will go away.

Increased thirst, which is also caused by water loss through increased urination

Sleep problems are very common during ketosis. Due to the lack of carbohydrates, the brain's normal function is disrupted. Levels of sleep-regulating neurotransmitters may also be disturbed for a time.

Feeling cold or having cold feet and hands. The low-carb diet that results in ketosis decreases thyroid function, thereby slowing metabolism and reducing body temperature.

Weakness caused by a lack of sufficient energy provided by carbohydrates.

Some people may experience nausea and vomiting. This is most likely the result of low sodium (hyponatremia) caused by increased water intake and urination. It's strongly recommended to make sure you get enough salt when in ketosis.

Reduced appetite is an extremely common side effect of ketosis, which is why it's an attractive option for weight-loss dieters.

The most definitive symptom is ketones in the urine. You can test for this by using ketone testing strips from you local drug store. If it turns purple, you're in ketosis.

THE ADVANTAGES AND DISADVANTAGES OF THE KETO DIET

Advantages of a Ketogenic Diet

In the past, low carb diets were considered to be unhealthy and many people believed that they contributed to high levels of cholesterol which led to heart diseases. Right after the turn of the millennium, scientists were able to show that low carb diets are very beneficial to human health.

Below are 5 advantages of ketogenic diet.

Helps with Weight Loss

Obesity is known to contribute to several complications such as hypertension and diabetes. Today, due to poor eating lifestyles and lack of exercising, many people are obese. In order to lose weight successfully, obese people need to engage in a low carb diet.

When an individual starts to consume low carb diets, the body helps to get rid of excess water which lowers insulin levels leading to the kidneys eliminating excess sodium and eventually weight loss. To ensure that you maintain a healthy body, it is important to consider low carb diets as a lifestyle and not as a diet.

Lows Risks of Hypertension

High blood pressure is a heart complication that occurs when fat is deposited around the walls of major blood vessels therefore narrowing the pathway. In this state, the heart uses a lot of pressure to pump blood through the narrowed vessels which eventually will lead to more heart complications.

Low carb diets help to eliminate or reduce the amount of saturated fats consumed. When low carb diets are consumed, the body utilizes the fat as energy in order to properly function. This helps to eliminate the fat in the vessels leading to a healthy life.

More Calories Are Burnt Efficiently

The human body is known to utilize more energy when burning fats. When one consumes low carb diets, the body helps to shed the excess fat stored around the thighs, waist and hips. As more calories are burnt, one will be able to perform strenuous activities with ease.

Increased Metabolism Rate

The digestion process is among the most complex functions in the body. Consumption of foods rich in saturated fats and high levels of carbs, will lower the metabolism leading to problems in bowel movement.

To ensure the metabolism rate increases, it is advisable to consume low carb diets as the body will be able to digest with ease.

Lowers Blood Sugar Levels

Consumption of low carb diets helps the body to convert them into simple sugars that are ingested by the body. When the body detects high glucose levels in the blood, it releases insulin which helps to direct the removal or storage of glucose.

By consuming low carb diets, the blood will have reduced levels of sugar.

Disadvantages of the Ketogenic Diet

The ketogenic diet was developed with the intention of introducing measured quantities of carbs, proteins and fats with the sole purpose of helping epileptic patients heal from their seizures. The success of the diet has led to its introduction in other areas such as weight loss. Although there are benefits, the ketogenic diet has disadvantages too.

Below are 5 disadvantages of the ketogenic diet.

Increases Risk of Heart Diseases

Low carb ketogenic diets are known to be high in saturated fats which usually increase the risk of heart diseases. Apart from high risk of heart diseases, there are other complications such as abdominal obesity as well as other obesity related disorders such as hypertension, diabetes and cancer.

Increases Chances of Weight Gain

Low carb diets usually promote increased fat burning meaning that the body will burn more than it is receiving. This means that when as an individual resorts to the normal intake of carbohydrates, the body will slow down in burning fat meaning it will increase your body weight.

Increases Chances of Ketosis

Due to the consumption of low carb diets, the body becomes severely restricted forcing the body to produce ketones in order to supply energy to areas of the body that don't use fat as an energy source. These areas include the brain and red blood cells.

The result of these is that an individual will be in a state of ketosis which is usually characterized by an acetone like smelly breath. Other effects include nausea and fatigue.

Intake of Low Nutrients

The body requires vital nutrients such as Vitamins, magnesium, potassium and calcium among others in order to function. Consumption of a low carb diet means that the body will lack vital nutrients therefore might lead to complications later.

Increased Chances of Muscle Breakdown

Consumption of low carb diets usually results in the body losing the water weight instead of fats. Prolonged consumption of this diet will eventually lead to the body breaking down muscles in order to utilize it as energy.

When one returns to a normal diet, the diet rebuilds the muscles and weight gain is experienced.

GETTING STARTED ON THE WEIGHT LOSS REGIME

List 5 Ways You Can Motivate Yourself to Lose Weight

1. Getting on the scale is one way to motivate you to lose weight. Those who avoid the scale on a regular basis, or don't go on the scale at all, are more than likely overweight. If you get on the scale, and see what your weight truly is, this can help to motivate you to lose weight right away.

2. If you have a disease related to your weight gain, this is a great motivator to lose weight. Diabetes, high blood pressure, high cholesterol, and other diseases can directly be linked to weight gain. If you contracted a weight related disease, or have weight related issues, learning about them can be a way to motivate you to lose weight.

3. A deadly diagnosis by a doctor linked to your weight, such as obesity should make you want to lose weight. Those who are morbidly obese are considered to be so overweight that they can actually die from it. If a doctor gives you this type of diagnosis, you need to lose weight as soon as possible. The will to live should be your only motivator to lose weight, because you may lose your life if you don't.

4. Think of the benefits of potential weight loss. If you're currently overweight, imagining yourself thin, as well as the health benefits, can help to motivate you to lose weight. Many lose weight for different reasons, but if you imagine yourself in a different light than you are in now, this can be a great way to motivate yourself to lose weight.

5. Keeping a daily food journal as well as keeping track of your weight, may motivate you to lose weight as well. If you see that certain foods you eat on a regular basis are making you gain weight, you may be motivated to lose weight by keeping and reading your food journal.

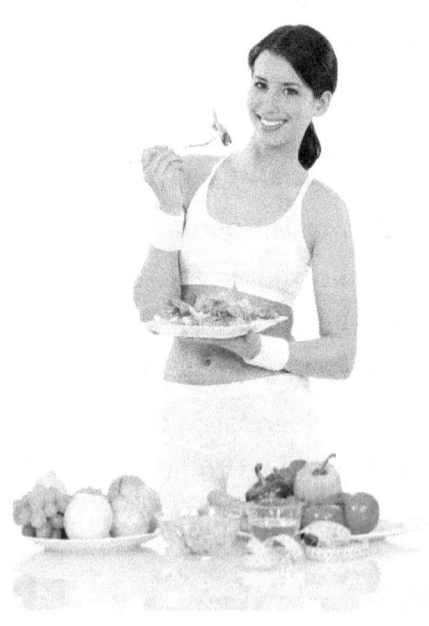

Exercise To Burn 1,000 Calories per Day and How to Do Them

1. If you want to burn 1000 calories in a day, an Elliptical machine can help you to do this. An Elliptical machine can be expensive, but the benefits that they give up make the price worth it. An Elliptical can help you burn up to 1000 calories in an hour if you continue at a steady pace. You may be able to burn even more than 1000 calories in an hour, if you decide to up the pace on the machine.

An Elliptical machine is fairly easy to use; you just step onto it with both feet, while holding on to the handlebars. Both the handlebars and the stands where you put your feet should be able to move simultaneously. Because this machine works the arms and legs, as well as the entire body at the same time, it quickly burns calories. Many diet and exercise experts out there recommend this machine when you want to lose weight quickly.

2. Running is another great way to burn 1000 calories in a day, but if you run at 7 mph, you can burn the thousand calories in an hour. If you're looking to burn 1000 calories over the course of a day, you can perform running several times throughout the day, depending on the amount of time that you have available. If you don't want to run one hour straight, break up your day into five different slots, and run 20 minutes each time.

If you have as little as two times in the day that you're available to run, perform two half-hour sets. Always take water with you when you are running for a long period of time, such as an hour. If you cannot bring water with you, make sure to stop somewhere along the way and replenish your body with water. Pace yourself when running, and stop if you begin to feel too much pain.

EAT THIS NOT THAT – FOODS YOU NEED AND DON'T NEED ON THE KETO DIET

Eating Daily to Consume 1500 Calories

Breakfast- when you're watching your calorie intake, you'll want to start out with a smoothie in the morning, in order to pace yourself to get to 1500 calories for the day. A smoothie should consist of yogurt, milk, and fruit. You can use alternative sweeteners to keep the calorie content lower, but try to avoid sugar. You'll get about 250 calories from your smoothie, depending on the foods you use in it.

Snack- After you've had your breakfast in the morning, you'll be hungry in a few hours, so add a snack of an Apple, which can also be taken with some pistachio nuts. If you combine the small apple with about 20 of the nuts, you'll have about 150 calories.

Lunch- Eat a salad that is mixed with lettuce, vegetables, raisins, almonds, a hard-boiled egg, and balsamic dressing. Keep the lettuce at 2 cups; add 1 cup of vegetables, and 2 teaspoons of all other ingredients. You can cut up the egg how you feel, and add it to your salad. This salad will be about 400 calories of your daily intake value.

Afternoon Snack- You can have one cup of carrot sticks, with hummus, or you can use low calorie ranch dressing. This type of snack can be fulfilling for the time being, and is about 150 calories.

Dinner- Make a homemade chicken pot pie that is creamy and filled with vegetables. You can find several recipes for this food, and if it's made correctly, it is very low in calories. The chicken you should add it to this pie is chicken breasts, as it has a lower calorie amount than any other part of the chicken. You'll also want to have a basic salad with your food, which consists of lettuce, red onions, and vinaigrette. This delicious dinner is about 500 calories, which will take you close to your 1500 calorie goal.

Eat These Superfoods That Help to Boost Metabolism and Weight Loss

If you are what you eat, then it goes without saying that what you put into your body should have a positive overall purpose. For those who are looking to help their skin's overall health, they should look to foods that are known for boosting circulation and skin healing. As for those who are hoping to boost their metabolism for the purpose of losing weight or getting fit, there are certain foods that can help you out in that area as well. The following list includes five super foods that are known to boost the metabolism and improve your overall daily eating regimen.

Lean Meats and Other Protein

With lean proteins, such as poultry and certain types of fresh water fish or seafood, you are introducing essential meats to your body that lack a lot of fat. Things like turkey or chicken require the body to digest with more effort than usual, which in turn speeds up the metabolism to accomplish a total breakdown of the food. There have been numerous studies to suggest that those who follow a high protein diet can burn twice as many calories as those who prefer a diet higher in carbohydrates.

Citrus

Everyone knows that a diet rich in Vitamin C is great for the body's overall function. Not everybody knows that foods like grapefruit, oranges, and lemons also give your body that extra boost of metabolism. Coupled with a decent workout regimen, eating citrus foods can boost your fat burn by up to forty percent.

Garlic

This herb has been used for many purposes throughout the years, but not many people realize just how much impact garlic can have on your metabolism. Garlic is believed to help the body shed pounds by allowing you to burn more calories in day to day activities.

Fiber Rich Fruits

Fruits that have plenty of fiber, such as berries, allow the body to work harder to digest. This boosts your metabolism rate. Since berries have very little calories per handful, this also makes for a wonderful snack to reach for during those moments where you crave something sweet.

Fiber Rich Cereals

There is a reason that athletes turn to cereals and other grains that are high in fiber and low in calories. Those who choose cereals with a lot of fiber for breakfast are a lot more likely to lose weight and be fit, than those who go for sugary cereals with little to no fiber.

Good & Bad Fats

Diet and good eating habits is the key to better health and better living. This is why one needs to know the differences between some common food components. This type of knowledge helps one make far better food choices and thus helps in overall better eating habits. The three fats that tend to confuse people are saturated fat, monounsaturated fat and polyunsaturated fat. They are all fats but they are all different.

Saturated fats are the ones that can be easily recognized simply by sight. They turn to a solid state when not heated and are at room temperature. Some of the most common saturated fats include butter, margarine and coconut oil. These are fats that can clog arteries and as such are not a wise dietary choice to be used all the time. Saturated fats should be used in moderation and avoided when possible. These fats are the traditional ones that were dietary staples for many years until people started realizing how bad they were for heart health and cholesterol levels.

Monounsaturated fats rank at the top of list of healthy fats and come from plants and animals. The common options are olive oil, preferably first cold pressed, sesame oil and canola oil. They are not as high in fatty acid and can be used on a routine basis for cooking, salad dressings, grilling, sautéing and even baking; provided they are used in moderation. These fats help lower bad cholesterol levels.

Polyunsaturated fats are derived from plants and tend to be the healthiest of the fats. They are known for lowering cholesterol levels that may have been elevated over time by eating too many saturated fats. Polyunsaturated fats that are used the most often and preferred for their taste include sunflower oil, soybean oil, cottonseed oil, safflower oil and corn oil. Polyunsaturated fats and oils are also ideal for both cooking and baking in a healthier manner compared to using fatty acids that are part of the saturated fats group.

Benefits of Omega-3 Fatty Oils

There are numerous health benefits associated with ingestion of the various omega-3 fatty oils found in many cold-water fish species. Five of the most important of these benefits are listed below.

1. Omega-3 Oils Can Have a Positive Effect on Cardiovascular Health

While studies sometimes conflict in their results and much more research needs to be done, there is good evidence that omega-3 oils help promote cardiovascular health. DHA and EPA, two of the most common omega-3 fatty acids, may reduce blood pressure, increase blood circulation, aid in combating varicose veins, and reduce the risk of heart attacks and strokes.

2. Omega-3 Can Fight Back Against Inflammations

Some studies have shown that the joint swelling, pain, and morning stiffness that come with having rheumatoid arthritis can be ameliorated by use of long-chain omega-3 oils. Consistent use over a period of several months may offer significant aid to those suffering with these sorts of inflammations.

3. Omega-3 Oils Can Help Combat Depression

Omega-3 fatty acids, particularly EPA, have been shown to have a positive impact on those suffering from bi-polar disorder and depression. Many of these fish oils are, in fact, widely considered to be beneficial to general mental health.

4. Omega-3 Can Provide Support for One's Ability to Recall Things

Diminishing of memory skills is a natural result of the aging process. However, there is clinical evidence to support the claim that omega-3 oils slow the onset of dementia or other memory problems. These oils are rich in nutrients that are needed by the brain for optimal cognition processes, and by getting sufficient quantities of omega-3, one may be able to retain his or her memory recall functions for longer in life.

5. Omega-3 Acids Increase Metabolism and Make Excellent Dietary Supplements

Many omega-3 fatty acids, especially DHA and EPA, are needed by the body for its everyday metabolic processes. Since these are rare elements in most modern diets, however, it is often important to take an omega-3 supplement.

Fish & the Ketogenic Diet

Aside from being a colorful and tasty asset to dining and cuisine, fish has been proven to have many health benefits. It is packed with vitamins and minerals. It is rich in protein and omega-3 fatty acids and low in fat. Eating one to two servings of fish a week can be a great boost to overall health. Let us list some of the specific benefits of eating fish.

Fish consumption can reduce the rate of heart disease and heart attack. When substituted for other foods containing saturated fats, eating fish can lower high cholesterol levels. Omega-3 fatty acids are also proven to decrease blood clotting and lower blood pressure, both blood clots and high blood pressure being precursors of heart disease.

Fish is brain food. Omega-3 is crucial for brain development, as much of the brain is actually made up of this type of fat. Children who eat fish regularly show better concentration skills and have a longer attention span. Regular consumption of fish has also been linked to fewer cases of dementia. Eating fish can lower the risk of depression as well since depression has been linked with an omega-3 deficiency in the brain.

Are you suffering from poor eyesight? A recent study showed that omega-3 helps to strengthen the retina of the eye. The large amounts of Vitamin A present in fish is also responsible for healthy eyes.

Omega-3 is a natural skin remedy. It is used to treat skin conditions such as eczema and psoriasis. The high quantities of protein in fish help produce skin collagen, which is needed for smooth, healthy skin.

Studies of populations that eat fish often found that those populations have very few cases of rheumatoid arthritis. There are those that suggest that Omega-3 fatty acids can actually relieve the symptoms of arthritis.

If you are not yet a fish fan, try to begin by substituting one meat meal a week for fish. You may find yourself to be a fan sooner than you expected.

Benefits of Eating Red and White Meat

The debate of whether red meat is bad or white meat is good for your health has been around for quite a while. What many people do not know is that both types of meats contribute significant amounts of nutrients to the body.

Below are 5 benefits of eating white and red meat.

Contribution of Iron in the Blood

Red meat is known to be a rich source of iron which forms the building blocks of blood and muscle function. It is vital in the body since it helps in the transportation of oxygen around the body. Antioxidant enzymes namely catalase and peroxidase helps to protect the cells from oxidation damage.

Another important function of iron in the body is that it helps the thyroid gland and the central nervous system to function properly.

Both Contain a Low Amount of Calories

Consumption of both red and white meat is known to contribute a low amount of calories in the body. While many people may believe that red meat contains more calories than white meat, the difference is quite negligible. Therefore you don't have to worry about spoiling your waistline when you consume red meat.

Provides Vitamin D to the Body

Vitamin D is a vital nutrient to the body as it helps in the absorption of calcium from foods. Apart from that, it helps in strengthening the teeth and bones. It is important to note that without Vitamin D, the body would be excreting calcium and it would not have been useful. Although the sun acts as an alternative source of Vitamin D, it also increases the rate of skin cancer.

Rich Source of Magnesium

Magnesium is an important nutrient in the body and it is required in huge amounts by each and every organ in the body. It helps to improve the proper functioning of the brain, the nervous system, the cardiovascular system, increases bone strength and muscles among others.

Consumption of meat which is rich in magnesium will enable the body gain huge quantities which will contribute to generation and use of ATP which is the fundamental unit of energy.

Rich Source of Vitamin B12

Vitamin B12 plays a vital role in the body as it helps in the formation of red blood cells. It also contributes to the formation of DNA and ensures that cells work efficiently. It is important to know that deficiency of Vitamin B12 can lead to dementia, loss of memory, anemia, fatigue, weakness and loss of appetite among others.

Spinach and Kale – Essential Foods for the Ketogenic Diet

Vegetables such as spinach and kale offer a variety of natural health benefits to the eater. Whether the healthful nutrients contained in these plants are ingested by consuming the plants themselves or through supplementation, one can expect positive results.

1. Spinach and many other green, leafy vegetables are rich in iron.

Iron is a necessary component of the hemoglobin in our blood, and many bodily enzymes and proteins require trace amounts of iron to perform optimally. Blood donors, small children, and pregnant women are especially at risk of iron deficiency. This mineral is so important that it is often used to enrich bread and breakfast cereals.

2. Kale and spinach are rich in vitamin K.

Kale especially, but spinach also, is extremely rich in vitamin K. Collard greens, Swiss chard, and mustard greens are other major sources. Vitamin K consumption is associated with bone health and a lower risk of diabetes in the elderly. It may also help reduce risk of coronary heart disease and some forms of cancer, but more research is needed.

3. Indole-3 carbinol is abundant in brassica vegetables.

Brassica vegetables, like kale and broccoli, are high in indole-3 carbinol, which boosts the ability of DNA to repair itself. This element may also block the growth of certain kinds of cancer cells.

4. Many leafy vegetables are high in vitamin A.

Spinach and many other leafy vegetables are high in vitamin A, which plays a wide variety of roles in maintaining bodily health. Vision, skin health, bone metabolism, immune system optimization, genetic transcription, and antioxidant activities all utilize vitamin A.

5. Kale and many brassicas contain abundant sulforaphane.

Sulphoraphane is a chemical found in kale and other vegetables that has been shown to possess powerful cancer-fighting abilities. It also works hard against neuro-degenerative diseases and is a potent antioxidant.

These five above-listed elements are only a portion of the many beneficial nutrients found in leafy vegetables. Many of these nutrients have multiple positive effects.

Dairy Products Such As Cheese and Sour Cream Are Staple On the Ketogenic Diet

1. Eating dairy products can be great for you, because some contain both calcium and protein. Calcium is great for building up bones, especially in children. Protein is good for building up muscle, and it helps you to feel fuller when you eat products containing protein. Protein is also recommended after exercising to help rebuild muscle, when it's used strenuously in exercising such as strength training.

2. Certain dairy products have Vitamin D in them, and others add Vitamin D to accommodate those who need

it. Vitamin D is good for helping to absorb calcium, and great for healthy bones. Vitamin D has also been known to help prevent cancers, and it's also good for lowering blood pressure. When choosing dairy products, it's best to pick the ones that contain Vitamin D.

3. Bone density is one benefit of eating dairy products. Calcium does help to build up bones, and this is found within many dairy products. It's best to get your calcium from dairy products as opposed to a pill form, because it's proven to give you denser bones. A study was performed on those who ate dairy products, and those who took calcium pills; dairy eaters had denser bones.

4. Dairy products have proven benefits to lower your blood pressure. Milk is great in the fight against high blood pressure, and drinking it on a daily basis gives you a 54% less chance of developing high blood pressure, if it's taken on a regular basis over a two-year period or longer.

5. Adding dairy products to your daily diet can lead to weight stabilization. Because many people can have their weight fluctuate up and down, those looking to regulate their weight should eat dairy products on a regular basis. Although it has not been proven that eating dairy products leads to higher weight loss, the calcium can help to stabilize your weight if eaten regularly.

Spices That Can Be Consumed When On a Ketogenic Diet

Low carb cooking and eating for those who are trying to remove carbohydrates from their diet often use a variety of spices to season foods. The majority of spices alone are low carb and thus most can be used to enhance the flavor of dishes, but, there are some spices that truly work wonders when maintaining a low carb diet.

Cayenne Pepper

Garlic

Cinnamon

Ginger

Cayenne pepper tops the list as a great addition to any low cab diet. The hot and spicy flavor adds a kick to any dish and the heat level can easily be adjusted by using more or less. In spice form, the cayenne pepper can add a touch of flavor and spiciness to foods such as steamed vegetables or any grilled protein. Cayenne pepper also has antioxidant and weight loss properties making it even better for those eating healthy.

Garlic has many beneficial qualities, from helping to boost immunity to being helpful in regulating glucose levels in the blood. The flavor of garlic is distinct, yet is pairs perfectly with just about any low carb dish. From salads and soups to meat and fish; garlic is one spice that works well for just about any savory dish.

Cinnamon has been known to have beneficial immunity boosting properties and it is a spice that has a smoky yet sweeter take. One can make low carb treats such as fresh berries or melon pop when cinnamon is used to flavor those low carb diet friendly dishes and desserts. Cinnamon can also be sprinkled on black tea or coffee for a boost of extra flavor that does not use refined sugar or dairy.

Ginger is a spice that has a very Eastern taste and offers plenty of healing qualities as well. Ginger is one spice that can enhance both sweet and savory dished and truly helps make low card eating more flavorful.

Do Not Eat Any Sugar

1. One of the biggest disadvantages to eating sugar is the fact that it can turn into fat in your body. Many did not realize that sugar made you gain weight, many believed that eating fat made you fat, or consuming many calories. It's been proven over time that this theory is untrue. If you wish to lose weight, or prevent gaining weight, you should cut sugar out of your diet as much as possible.

2. There are absolutely no vitamins or minerals in sugar, only empty calories. These empty calories can then make

you hungrier, and even make you crave more sugar. If you're looking for a diet that has vitamins and minerals, so you can eat healthier; sugar should not be a part of that diet, because it adds absolutely no value to your daily food intake. It's best to just avoid sugar altogether if possible.

3. Eating sugar can cause blood sugar spikes, which can be bad for anyone even if they do not have diabetes. Those with diabetes need to be most aware of their blood sugar, but those who are dieting should also be aware of their blood sugar as well. Having a spike in your blood sugar can make you crash later, causing hunger, weakness, and tiredness.

4. Sugar is the cause of several diseases, including Obesity, Diabetes, and Heart Disease. Eating large amounts of sugar can lead to weight gain, and gaining too much weight can then lead to obesity. Certain Diabetes is also caused by the over consumption of sugar over time. Eating sugar can eventually lead to Heart Disease as well.

5. Sugar can be extremely addictive to some people. Although it has yet to be proven to be physically addictive, it's proven to be psychologically addictive. Dopamine is released in the brain when you consume sugar, leading to feelings of pleasure. It's believed that sugar has addictive properties similar to drugs.

Do Not Eat Any Grains

Foods made from wheat have been advertised as contributors to the well being of the human body. What many people don't know is that wheat by products has a negative impact to human health.

Below are 5 disadvantages of consuming/eating grains such as wheat.

Increases Blood Sugar Level

Foods made from wheat are usually broken down into glucose and then absorbed into the blood. These usually results in increase of blood sugar which prompts the body to release insulin. Insulin helps to eliminate and also direct the storage of glucose in cells. Increase in blood sugar leads to generation of free radicals which cause damage to cells too.

Increases Insulin Levels Leading To Complications

Insulin is produced by the pancreas to help counteract the high levels of blood sugar. High insulin levels have been found to contribute to several complications such as obesity, high blood pressure, diabetes, heart disease, dementia and some forms of cancer.

Low Quantity of Useful Nutrients

Nutrients are very vital in the body as they help in the running and nutrition of organs in the body. Wheat products have been found to contribute nutrients which are barren of fiber. This means that less or no useful nutrients are contributed when one consumes wheat products.

Increases Allergic Reactions

Many people are allergic to gluten which is found in wheat products. Allergic reactions to gluten usually lead to several complications and immediate medical response is required.

Wheat Products Contain Lectins

Lectins found in wheat products usually elevate gut permeability therefore leading to introduction of junk into the blood. The immune system usually gets confused between the junk and the body proteins since they look similar. This results in the immune system attacking both the junk and the proteins and may lead to several complications like acne and sclerosis.

Do Not Eat Any Corn Produced Products

1. Although corn is a vegetable and normally good for you, most corn today is genetically modified. Genetically modified corn is great at keeping away pests, and giving a greater yield, which lowers the cost and increases the

profit for farmers. The problem with genetically modified corn is that there is no telling what the long-term effects can be on humans, or on their health. Because genetically modified corn can kill pests that consume it, the theory is, it may also be harmful to humans as well. Up to 85% of corn today is genetically modified.

2. Cornstarch is a derivative of corn, and is used to thicken foods such as soups, gravies, and sauces. The problem with this product is that it can turn to sugar in the body, which can then be stored as fat. It's also high in carbohydrates, and too much of it can lead to weight gain.

3. Corn syrup is used to sweeten many different foods including candy. Even with the use of this product, it can contribute to many health issues including weight gain, high blood sugar, and diabetes. You can find this product in a different form called high fructose corn syrup, which is in many products such as yogurt, soda, fruit drinks and more. This additive to foods, directly contributes to weight gain, as well as diabetes.

4. Corn that is created today causes allergies in many who consume it, although this is unknown to the consumer. Corn is processed into many different foods, and the corn content in the food can cause allergies in some people. Some may attribute the symptoms to something other than corn, until a diagnosis from a doctor proves otherwise.

5. Corn is added to hundreds of products after being processed. Many eat corn every day and don't know it, and it contributes to their poor overall health, including excessive weight, and several diseases.

Do Not Eat Starchy Foods

1. Starchy foods can have empty calories, which provide no nutrients, and can lead you to feeling hungry quicker. When you eat certain starchy foods such as bread, pizza, or other items with flour, you are getting empty calories that are high in carbohydrates. Starchy foods can make you feel hungry faster than you normally would, if you consume these types of foods.

2. Starchy foods are full of carbohydrates, which can lead to weight gain. Depending on the amount of starchy foods you eat, and what type you eat, you may end up gaining weight, especially when eating flour products. Those who are on a low-carb diet should avoid starchy foods, because the carbs will not allow you to lose weight efficiently, and starchy foods are packed full of carbs.

3. Starchy foods make it hard for you to lose weight when you include them in any diet. Although you can add certain starchy foods such as fruits and potatoes to your diet, others, such as pasta, pizza, and bread are not recommended. The carbohydrates in starchy foods can

help you to pack on the pounds, and the sugar in them can be turned to fat in your body.

4. Many starchy foods contain sugar content, and this can contribute to weight gain, blood sugar problems, as well as diabetes. Those who are looking to lead a healthier life need to cut out starchy foods as much as possible, because of the negative overall impact on the body, and because of the sugar content.

5. When eating starchy foods that are fried, you are contributing to your bad cholesterol, which is bad for your overall health. Frying starchy foods such as tortillas, doughnuts, fillets, and potato chips can lead to extra calories, which in turn, can lead to weight gain, heart attack, and a buildup of bad cholesterol in the body.

Do Not Eat Processed Foods

1. Processed foods are full of sodium. It's recommended that you eat 2000 mg of sodium per day, and some processed foods have that amount in one serving. The excessive salt that is in processed foods can lead to high blood pressure. The high sodium amount in these foods is to prevent bacteria growth, but it, in turn, makes the product less healthy for those who consume it.

2. Processed foods may contain refined grains, which can lead to weight gain, and obesity. When processors refine grains, they take out the good nutrition, and only leave

the unessential nutrients just to preserve the shelf life of the product. Refined grains introduced into society hundreds of years ago, have contributed to poor health, as well as a lower average height in humans who eat these products.

3. Trans fats can be found in processed foods, although many places have outlawed adding them to foods. Trans fats will help to prolong the shelf life of a processed food, but it contributes to many health problems in humans. Trans fats also can raise the level of bad blood pressure that you have, while lowering your good blood pressure.

4. Studies have shown that IQ in children, who eat processed foods from the age of three, can be lowered considerably. In the same studies, children who ate a balanced diet had a better IQ than those who ate processed foods regularly. It's best to provide children with a healthy balanced diet of whole foods, and to avoid processed foods as much as possible.

5. It's a known fact that processed foods can make you gain weight, which is a great disadvantage. Although processed foods are usually cheaper, taste better, and last longer, they are bad for the body. It may be tempting to reach for these items when you want something to eat, but you may want to consider your waistline.

Do Not Eat Fruits

Fruit is healthy for you, this is true. Do not assume, though, that you can consume a massive amount of fruit and not suffer any ill-effects. Here are five legitimate disadvantages to eating fruit.

Fruit Can Make You Fat

This might seem like a shocking assessment since fruit is a staple of good diets. True, fruit is low in calories and has no saturated fats. The trouble is fruit is loaded with sugar. If you consumer too much sugar, even natural sugar, you end up with a lot of glucose in the bloodstream. All that glucose is going to turn to fat if it is not burned.

Fruit Might Contribute to Hyperactivity

This is another byproduct of the excess sugar found in fruit. Sugar creates energy which can be a good thing in moderation. When your energy levels are so high you become hyperactive, this is not a positive thing. In fact, excess hyperactivity could create anxiety and lead to social problems.

Not a Source of Protein

Your body needs to have a healthy supply of protein in its diet in order to maintain and repair muscle mass. Protein also aids in ensuring the metabolism works properly and you maintain a lean physique. Eating fruit at the exclusion of foods with protein could create a deficiency.

Too Much of Certain Vitamins

There is such a thing as having too much of a single vitamin. Eating citrus fruit to excess, for example, might cause your body to ingest way more vitamin C than it should have or can process.

Too Much Sugar Could Lead to Diabetes

High sugar content in a diet can lead to problems with diabetes. You simply cannot maintain very high amounts of sugar in the bloodstream and not experience negative, debilitating effects as a result. The common refrain that natural sugar is good for you is not always correct. Too much sugar any kind of sugar, could lead to adverse health problems.

Do Not Drink Milk

1. A High Source of Calories in Milk

As far as beverages are concerned, milk is considered fairly high in calories. One cup of 1 percent milk contains approximately 103 calories. Drinking even a few glasses a day will dramatically increase caloric intake. Milk is not only relatively high in calories but loaded with saturated fat as well.

2. Lots of Hormones in Milk

A lot of dairy farmers include a variety of hormones in the diets of their cows. An increase in hormone levels could be related to a higher incidence of cancers including breast and prostate cancer. In particular, bovine growth hormones have been given to cows to help them produce more milk. The bovine hormone was approved for use in the US in 1993.

3. Not That Much Calcium in Milk

While there is calcium in milk, there's really not that much compared to other sources. Marketing campaigns have hyped the health benefits of drinking milk. Spinach, kale, and turnip greens all offer great sources of calcium that may be healthier overall to eat. Even oranges and sesame seeds can provide calcium in place of milk.

4. Cow's Milk Really Isn't for People

Yes, technically we can drink it, but milk that cow's make is better suited for other cows. The chemical and overall nutritional content of a cow's milk is basically for turning a newborn calf into a 400 pound adult cow in one year. This means that even though there are good nutrients in the milk, it contains more of certain minerals than what humans really need.

5. Lactose Intolerance

It's estimated that over 50 percent of adults have at least some difficulty digesting milk. People who are lactose intolerant can experience a variety of symptoms when drinking milk. A few of these can include nausea, diarrhea, bloating, and cramps.

ONE MONTH OF KETOGENIC RECIPES

KETOGENIC DIET BREAKFAST RECIPES

Yogurt, Spinach, Chili Oil Baked Eggs

Servings: 2-4

Calories: 223

Ingredients:

Plain Greek yogurt (2/3 c)

Garlic clove (1- halved)

Kosher salt (to taste)

Unsalted butter (2Tbs- divided)

Leek (3Tbs-chopped)

Scallion (2Tbs-chopped)

Spinach (10 0z)

Lemon juice (1 tsp)

Eggs (4)

Red pepper flakes (1/4 tsp)

Oregano (1 tsp)

Olive oil (2Tbs)

Instructions:

Combine yogurt, garlic, and salt. Preheat oven-300 degrees. Melt 1Tbs butter with oil in skillet. Add leek and scallion-cook until tender. Add spinach and lemon juice. Turn heat to medium-high and cook until spinach is wilted. Place spinach mixture in 10" skillet.

Make 4 indentations in the spinach. Add eggs to indentation. Bake 10-15 minutes. Melt the remaining butter. Add red pepper flakes to butter-cook 2 minutes. Add oregano and cook ½ minute. Remove garlic from yogurt. Spoon yogurt over eggs and top with butter.

Tofu Scramble

4-6 serving

390 calories

Ingredients:

Extra-firm tofu (2-14oz blocks)

Vegetable oil (2Tbs)

Small onion- chopped

Small bell pepper- finely chopped

Cumin (1/2 tsp)

Coriander (1/2 tsp)

Turmeric (1 1/2tsp)

Black beans (15 oz- drained, rinsed)

Cilantro (1/4 cup, chopped)

Salt, pepper

Wheat tortillas (4 to 6, warmed)

Instructions:

Smash tofu. Cook onion and peppers in oil. Add cumin and coriander. Cook 1 minute. Add tofu and turmeric. Add beans. Cook for 2 minutes, stir constantly. Add cilantro, salt, pepper.

Serve with tortillas.

Omar Peart

Quinoa Breakfast

Serves 4

Calories -492

Ingredients:

Quinoa (1 c)

Eggs (4)

Olive oil (2Tbs)

Avocado (1, chopped)

Smoked Salmon (6 oz)

Lemon juice and scallions (garnish)

Instructions:

Cook quinoa. Heat oil and add eggs.

Cover and cook eggs 2 to 4 minutes then season with salt and pepper.

Top quinoa with eggs, avocado, and salmon and garnish as desired.

Bacon and Eggs

6 servings

Calories – 204 per egg

Ingredients:

Cream cheese (3.5 oz)

Thyme (1/4 tsp)

Eggs (6, hard-boiled)

Bacon (12 slices)

Instructions:

Preheat oven -400 degrees. Combine cream cheese and thyme. Cut peeled eggs lengthwise. Remove yolks then fill 6 egg halves with cream cheese. Top with the other egg halves.

Tightly wrap each stuffed egg with two slices of bacon. Place eggs in shallow glass baking dish. Bake for 30 minutes.

Remove and serve.

KETOGENIC DIET LUNCH RECIPES

One can consume a hearty lunch, yet still keep their calorie intake in check by trying their hand at an Herbed Cheese and Tomato sandwich, Turkey Wrap, Spicy Black Bean Burrito, and a Grilled Cheese with Turkey and Tomato sandwich. Each is under 400 calories, but will provide the needed energy burst to get one through the second half of their day.

Herbed Cheese and Tomato

Ingredients:

English muffin toasted or untoasted

Low fat cottage cheese (1/4 cup)

Two slices of green or red tomato

A quarter of an avocado

Chopped chives (1 tbsp)

One leaf of butter lettuce

Brown mustard (1 tbsp)

Instructions:

Create the sandwich with an English muffin toasted or untoasted, while adding low fat cottage cheese (1/4 cup), two slices of green or red tomato, and slice a quarter of an avocado. Complete the sandwich with chopped chives (1 TBSP), one leaf of butter lettuce, and spice it up with brown mustard (1 TBSP). Add a banana for desert, and one stays well line with a 400 calorie lunch.

Turkey Wrap

Turkey is a choice many go to during their lunch hour, and a wrap is a quick source of protein while keeping calories in check.

Ingredients:

Whole wheat wrap

Three slices of lean deli turkey

Hummus (2 tbsp)

Goat cheese (1 tbsp)

Handful of baby spinach

Bag of Garlic and Herb Pita chips

Instructions:

The Turkey Wrap is put together with a whole wheat wrap, and three slices of lean deli turkey. Next add hummus to the wrap (2 TBSP), goat cheese (1 TBSP), and a generous handful of baby spinach. One can add a bag of Garlic and Herb Pita chips to the wrap to stay under 375 calories for this delectable lunch.

Grilled Turkey Sandwich with Cheese and Tomato

Ingredients:

Whole wheat bread (2 slices)

Lean deli turkey (3 slices)

Provolone cheese (1 slice)

Olive oil

Instructions:

A second turkey option is to add grilled cheese and tomato to the sandwich. Ensure the butter is left off of the whole wheat bread to keep this sandwich under 350 calories. The sandwich is created with two slices of whole wheat bread, and three slices of lean deli turkey. Add one slice of provolone cheese, toast it in a Panini press, and spritz some olive oil on the bread for taste. Add an apple for desert to finish off a healthy lunch alternative.

Bean Burrito

Ingredients:

Black beans (1/4 cup)

Whole wheat wrap

Quarter of an avocado

Red onion finely sliced

Mild, hot, or extra hot sauce (1 tspn)

10 or so baked tortilla chips

Quarter of a cup of salsa

Instructions:

Add black beans (1/4 cup) to a whole wheat wrap so one enjoys the fiber benefit of the lunch. Include a quarter of an avocado, and red onion finely sliced. Next to kick it up, use your favorite mild, hot, or extra hot sauce (1 TSPN). Finish off the lunch menu with 10 or so baked tortilla chips with a quarter of a cup of salsa. All four of these options provide one with the fuel needed to finish off the work day strong.

KETOGENIC DIET DINNER RECIPES

Arugula and Pear Salad Topped with Candied Walnuts (208 calories)

Ingredients:

Original Recipe:

Brown sugar candied walnuts (1 cup)

Garlic clove, large, minced (1)

Walnut oil (2 tbsp)

Dijon mustard (1 tbsp)

White wine vinegar (1 tbsp)

Ground pepper (1/4 tsp.)

Baby arugula (8 cups)

Red pears, ripe, sliced (2)

Instructions:

Put the salt and garlic in a bowl and mash together. Add to a large salad bowl to pepper, vinegar, mustard and oil. Then add the candied walnuts, pears and arugula.

Chile Relleno Mini Casserole (215 calories)

Ingredients:

Original Recipe:

Salt (1/4 tsp.)

Eggs, large (4)

Egg whites (6)

Non-fat milk (1 ½ cups)

Cheddar, reduced fat, shredded (1 cup)

Scallions, sliced thinly (4)

Frozen corn, thawed and dried (3/4 cup)

Green Chiles, diced, drained, dried (2 4 oz. cans)

Instructions:

Preheat the oven to 400F and use heatproof ramekins coating with cooking spray and baking sheet. Divide the scallions, corn and green Chiles equally among ramekin. Top with cheddar. Mix eggs, egg whites, salt and milk in a separate bowl and divide it evenly among all the ramekins. Bake for about 25 – 35 minutes, until the eggs are set and the top is browned.

Butternut Baja Squash Soup (55 calories)

Ingredients:

Original Recipe:

Chives of Parsley, chopped (2 tbsp)

Yoghurt, plain and non-fat (1/2 cup)

Ground pepper (1/4 tsp)

Sea salt (1 tsp)

Vegetable broth (6 cups)

Ground clove (1/8 tsp)

Ground cumin (1 tsp)

Chipotle (1/2 tsp)

Carrot, nicely chopped (1)

Onion, small, diced (1)

Celery stalks, chopped (2)

Canola oil (1 tsp)

Butternut (1 ½ lbs)

Instructions:

Preheat the oven to 350F. Bake the halved squashes and scoop the flesh out. In a saucepan, heat some oil and add carrot, onion and celery. Cook for about 10 minutes and add cloves, chipotle, cumin and squash. Add the vegetable broth and cook for 20 – 25 minutes. Puree and use pepper and salt to season.

Lettuce Leaf Tacos (550 calories)

Ingredients:

Original Recipe:

Green bell pepper, nicely chopped (1)

Yellow onion, nicely chopped (1)

Olive oil (2 tbsp)

Ground beef (1 lb)

Taco seasoning (3 tbsp)

Plum tomatoes, nicely chopped (2)

Salt (1/2 tsp)

Cheddar cheese, packaged, shredded (8 oz)

Romaine lettuce, large (12 leaves)

Instructions:

Cook yellow onion and bell pepper in olive oil for 5 minutes. In a separate pan, add ground beef and taco seasoning. Cook for 5 – 8 minutes till beef is crumbly. Add 2 tbsp. of beef filling to every lettuce leaf, top with 2 tsp. of pepper-onion mixture, tomatoes and 1 tbsp. cheddar cheese.

KETOGENIC DIET VEGETABLE SMOOTHIE RECIPES

Beetroot Spinach Almond Smoothie

Ingredients:

One cooked beet

One large apple, peeled and chopped

Half cup red grape juice

One cup washed spinach

One cup raw almond milk

Instructions:

Blend ingredients in blender till smooth for one minute. Serve immediately.

Beetroot Cherry Lettuce Smoothie

Ingredients:

One medium Beetroot, peeled and chopped

One cup cherries, seeded

Half cup hemp seeds

One cup romaine lettuce

One cup filtered water

Instructions:

Blend ingredients in blender for one minute till smooth. Serve immediately with chopped ice if desired.

Topical Green Smoothie

Ingredients:

One large ripe peeled banana

One fourth cup avocado

6 ounces fresh spinach

Three fourths cup pineapple

One cup frozen mango

Four ice cubes

One tablespoon coconut milk powder

One cup pure water

Instructions:

Pour water in a blender, adding additional ingredients in and blend till smooth one minute.

Spinach Peach Smoothie

Ingredients:

Six peaches, chopped

Six ounces fresh spinach

Two cups water

One tablespoon coconut milk powder

Instructions:

Pour in water, chopped peaches, spinach and coconut milk powder. Blend ingredients till smooth for one minute.

Omar Peart

Cherry Cabbage Smoothie

Ingredients:

Half cup orange juice

One cup frozen cherries

Half cup red cabbage

One teaspoon honey

One eighth teaspoon cinnamon

Four ice cubes

Instructions:

Chop ice cubes in a blender for twenty seconds. Then combine remaining ingredients with chopped ice and blend for one minute.

Winter Blueberries Smoothie

Ingredients:

Half cup frozen blueberries

Half cup avocado

Small peeled fresh banana

Six ounces kale

Two cups water

One tablespoon cocoa powder

One tablespoon raw honey

Pinch cayenne pepper

Instructions:

Blend ingredients until smooth.

Omar Peart

Broccoli and Spinach Apple Smoothie

Ingredients:

One finely chopped carrot

Four broccoli florets

8 ounces spinach

One chopped apple

Two oranges peeled

Two cups water

Instructions:

Blend ingredients until smooth.

Cucumber Mint Smoothie

Ingredients:

One cup coarsely chopped fresh cauliflower

One cup one-inch chopped honeydew melon

One half cup cucumber, cut into cubes

One half cup lightly packed fresh mint leaves

One fourth cup honey

Half cup ice cubes

Instructions:

In small pan, cook cauliflower uncovered for ten minutes. Drain into cold water. In a blender add cooked cauliflower, melon, cucumber, mint and honey and blend until smooth. Then add ice cubes and blend until smooth.

Omar Peart

Asparagus Smoothie

Ingredients:

Four ounces trimmed asparagus

Three cups fresh baby spinach

One cup seedless green grapes

Two kiwifruit, peeled and chopped

One half cup white grape juice

Three fourths cup ice cubes

Instructions:

Cook asparagus covered in boiling water five minutes till tender. Remove from heat, drain and cool five minutes.

Blend asparagus, spinach, grapes, kiwifruit and grape juice and blend till smooth. Add ice cubes and blend.

Mango Spinach Honey Smoothie

Ingredients:

One cup chopped fresh mango

One cup fresh spinach

Two tablespoons raw honey

Half cup orange juice

Four chopped ice cubes

Instructions:

In blender, add ingredients and blend one minute till smooth. Add ice cubes and blend additional twenty seconds till smooth. Serve immediately.

Omar Peart

www.ingramcontent.com/pod-product-compliance
Lightning Source LLC
Chambersburg PA
CBHW060640290526
45793CB00001B/329